Chakras:
How to Awaken Your Internal Energy through Chakra Meditation

Jen Solis

CONTENTS

Introduction

Conclusion

Introduction

I want to thank you and commend you for taking time to read the book, "Chakras".

How to Awaken Your Internal Energy through Chakra Meditation" .

This book contains a detailed overview of a truth that has long been hidden from us in the West. While modern science has brought us many fruits, mental wellbeing is not one of them. The ancients knew a deeper truth that allowed them to lead more fulfilled lives, at least in terms of their emotional and psychological wellbeing. We are going to teach you how to tap into that knowledge to bring about a quality of life you have always wanted. Perhaps you didn' t think it was possible. Maybe you think you don' t deserve happiness. Neither of these thing are true. True happiness, enlightenment, and clarity of purpose are possible. Better yet, *you* are deserving of such a wondrous fate. I will show you the secret techniques to channeling your inner energy and bringing forth your purpose.

So what can you expect? Well, nothing works unless you do. If you consistently engage in the practices outlined in this book, you will see results in your daily life. You will be able to diagnose the sources of issues that bother you, and take action to fix them for good. I would like to stress that there are no quick fixes, but after a few weeks of practice you will notice the first signs of results. If you stick with it for your lifetime, then you will become who you were destined to be.

Chapter 1
Everything You Ever Wanted to Know About Chakras, but Were Afraid to Ask.

All life is a balance between positive and negative energy. For humans, many of the conditions facing us (health, wellbeing, productivity, etc.) are determined by the energy balance in our bodies. These energies originate from and flow to different centers within the human body. Located all over the body, the function of each of the centers varies, as do the consequences for imbalances. When people talk about chakras, it is these centers they are referring to.

Most of us are familiar with the consequences of energetic imbalances. We may feel groggy, unmotivated, even depressed. These are, of course, the consequences of an imbalance of negative energy. The flip side, feeling healthy, motivated, and energetic is a consequence of an excess of positive energies within the chakras. What is missing in Western thought is the ancient origins of this phenomenon. The ancients were familiar with this, as it is a fundamental facet of the human experience, but their understanding transcended the mere observational. They didn't simply contemplate the sensations coursing through their body. The ancients (in the East) made a number of deductions about the phenomenon.

Modern man has taken a different route to managing these energetic imbalances. Modern medicine has done wonders for improving our longevity. This book won't argue that you should stop taking antibiotics for bacterial infections. Rather, what we are going to argue is that many psychological afflictions have a more fundamental cause in our own energetic system. While you should rely on modern medicine for treatment of grave physical conditions, the treatment of psychological distress should rely on more holistic and Eastern methods.

These methods will take the form of meditations and visualizations that will help you redirect your energies to "unclog" the energy and allow it to flow more freely. This will let the negative energy to flow out, and the positive to flow in. Just like a sink eventually becomes revolting if you leave it clogged long enough, you can suffer psychological harm from a long term imbalance of energies. Fortunately, this damage is not permanent.

Since we know that chakras are the energy centers of the body, it is reasonable to ask: where are they located? Great question! Let's take a basic tour of the human body with an eye for the locations of the various chakras. We'll get to the meat of how to use this information to make lasting and positive changes in your life in a later chapter.

Root Chakra:

It makes sense to start with the root chakra. Out of all the chakras in your body, this one is the most "physical". It is related to the basic physical needs of our survival. Things like food, water, shelter, comfort, and our personal finances. Yes, even the money in your pocket is related to a chakra.

When your environment is abundant in the necessities, your root chakra is fulfilled. When you are living in an environment of scarcity, the root chakra is lacking. Manipulation of the flow of energy through the root chakra is what will help you to improve your overall physical situation in life.

Sacral Chakra:

The second stop on our journey through the chakras is the sacral. It is located right below your belly button (navel). The sacral chakra is associated with our feelings and emotions. It's rather sad that in Western society we are taught to suppress emotions, particularly those that are negative.

As an aside, this afflicts both genders. Women are taught to be pleasant and not rock the boat. They are taught to not assert themselves in social situations. Men are taught to not show emotion, other than anger. It is unacceptable for men to demonstrate affection and kindness, as it is seen as weakness. The consequence of this is a Los Angeles rush hour-sized imbalance in the sacral chakra.

Fixing this imbalance can result in a freer flow of emotion. This takes the form of letting go of baggage, ceasing the practice of living in the past, and really living in the joy of the moment. The consequences of clearing out your sacral chakra are truly far reaching in your life.

One thing that will improve is emotional intimacy. If you are having difficulty in your relationships, a lack of intimacy can be a cause or an effect. Either way, fixing the energy imbalance in this chakra will be a positive step towards improving the intimacy in your personal relationships.

Solar Plexus Chakra:

Moving on up the body, we arrive at the solar plexus. This is located just below the heart, to right above the navel. The solar plexus chakra is the energetic center of our ego, our sense of self, and our self-esteem. Many of us are going to struggle with imbalances here, with a variety of consequences.

Feelings of inadequacy are common, particularly in a society where we are constantly exposed to sterling examples of beauty in the media. Women are regularly exposed to photoshopped images of celebrity women. This sets up an unattainable standard, resulting in feelings of inadequacy and a lack of self-esteem. This results in an energetic mess at the solar plexus, and it often spills over into the rest of our lives.

For men, issues with the solar plexus chakra can manifest in feelings of powerlessness. In the West there is a growing feeling of powerlessness amongst men, as evidenced by the popularity and rise of divisive and extremist politicians. The popularity of people who tell us there is a problem and it's not our fault is a direct manifestation of rampant feelings of powerlessness. It turns out that our energetic imbalances at the individual level can result in surprising phenomena at the social level.

Another consequence is a lack of confidence and follow through. Many of us have imposter syndrome when we achieve success. We feel like we are fakers, or that we don't deserve to be successful. This results in self sabotage and an eventual monumental blow up.

Fixing the imbalance in the solar plexus chakra is going to be the key to getting your professional life on track. If you find yourself lacking the power to start ambitious new projects, you're going to want to pay special attention to the instructions for clearing out the imbalances in your solar plexus.

Heart Chakra:

Our next stop is the heart chakra. While many of us associate the heart with the sensation of love, the heart chakra is involved in much deeper facets of our psyche. Of course, the sacral chakra is responsible for our emotional wellbeing, so what function does the heart chakra serve?

The heart chakra is involved in our ability to feel empathy and sympathy for other human beings. These are the qualities of being able to see the lives of someone else in our own. When another person is going through a rough time, it causes us to experience emotions that are identical to what we would experience in the same situation. This is because we empathize with them, meaning that we can picture ourselves in their shoes.

Empathy is the root cause of many of our social institutions. Most people are decent because it makes us feel bad to do harmful things to other people. Of course, society likes to beat this quality out of us because it serves the purposes of the authorities. It is difficult to get empathetic people to go to war, or to support a war. It is difficult to get empathetic people to turn away desperate refugees. Rather, we are taught that our lives and feelings are more important as a consequence of an accident of birth (i.e. where you are born).

While I have waxed political a little bit, it is to make a point. The lack of empathy in the individual has far reaching consequences. If you aren't as concerned with the consequences for other people, then this is a symptom of an imbalance in your heart chakra.

The consequences of this are quite personal, not just political. A lack empathy leads to discord in our own personal relationships. It is difficult to engage in constructive debate with a spouse if you are incapable of seeing their point of view – both emotionally and logically. Fixing the energy imbalance in the heart chakra is going to be key to improving your personal life, as well as improving society as a whole. Alas, you can't control the behavior of others, but you can certainly lead by example.

Throat Chakra:

Continuing up the body we arrive at the throat. As the voice box is associated with verbal communication, the throat chakra is likewise concerned with expressing yourself. This isn't just limited to speech. It encompasses art, body language, and other forms of communication.

It is helpful to think of the chakras as a sort of building. Each one rests upon the one below it, and builds upon its qualities. If your lower chakras are in balance, then the throat chakra will allow you to speak truth. You will articulate what is in your heart, your mind, and your deepest thoughts.

This may seem somewhat inconsequential, but I would invite you to reconsider. How many times have you sat down to talk with someone and gotten the feeling they weren't genuine? What effect did this have on your perception of them? Many times, this can be a warning sign that something isn't right. Those that are hiding something negative will often have an imbalance of energy, and this results in a blockage before the throat chakra. This manifests itself as communication that broadcasts the imbalance. They may be saying the right words, but something is off.

Focus on taking care of your lower chakras and you will not fall prey to this pitfall. You will be genuine and sincere in everything you say. Those around you will appreciate this, and you will find that your social status skyrockets. Everybody likes genuine people, and nobody likes a faker.

Third Eye Chakra:

We've now arrived at your head. As you might expect, we're getting close to the end of our journey. However, the third eye chakra is one of the most important in your social interactions. The third eye governs our intuition, and it is the third eye that allows us to see through the façade of a liar.

In the section on the throat chakra, I spoke of being able to sense when someone isn't genuine. This is a consequence of having a finely tuned third eye chakra. It allows you to see beyond what is right in front of you to understand more than meets the physical eye. The third eye is our source of intuition, and it is truly critical for our life.

Not only is it involved with seeing the truth in others, it is also involved in divining universal truths. Those that can make extrapolations beyond the here and now have a strong third eye. By this I mean what the West would call inductive reasoning. It is the ability to generalize from past experience into future predictions. This is a form of intelligence, of course. Those that have what many consider a powerful intellect have a highly active and powerful third eye chakra.

If you've ever found yourself unable to determine the right path in life, then that is probably a result of an imbalance in your third eye. When you are confronted with multiple possibilities but are unable to see which is the best, something isn't quite right. For those that have a highly functional third eye, indecision isn't a problem. Second guessing isn't a problem. They know they are making the right choice, because they can see beyond what is right in front of them into the consequences of their actions. We may call this a highly advanced ability to simulate the future, in the parlance of the scientific traditions of Western civilization.

Needless to say, you will want to develop this chakra and be sure to keep it clear of imbalances. In doing so, you will lead a more fulfilling life, because you will know the right choice in every situation. You will be able to reason from first principles, meaning that you will take what you *know* to be true and use that to make decisions. By this, I mean that you will take certain things to be true and make decisions based on that knowledge. If you believe stealing is wrong, you don't have to ponder whether or not you should rob your neighbor while they are on vacation.

The Crown Chakra:

You may have thought we had nowhere to go once we hit the third eye. That's not quite right, as it turns out. The final stop is at the culmination of all that has preceded it. At the very top of the head is the crown chakra, and it serves a marvelous purpose.

It is the hub of all the chakras below it, and serves as a sort of integrator. It brings it all together. But it doesn't just bring together the energies of the individual, it connects them to the universal consciousness. The world's great religious thinkers and prophets have had especially powerful crown chakras. This enabled them to see divine truth and achieve a connection with the higher power.

For those of us who don't want to become the next great spiritual leader, there is still utility in cleansing the crown chakra. Integrating all the energy from the underlying chakras is truly powerful, and can have surprising results in your life. The greatest leaders, both in deeds and in thought, have well-developed and clear crown chakras.

Through development of your crown chakra you will become a living manifestation of your purpose. If you are on a mission to help one million people achieve their dreams, and you are living that dream every moment of every day that is a manifestation of the crown chakra. Tony Robbins is one example of this in Western culture. His self-help books and seminars have helped legions of people achieve their potential. He does this through actualizing *his own* full potential and leading by example. He is but one example, and probably not even the best.

It is also involved in being able to see the big picture. If you've ever sat down and contemplated how seemingly inconsequential facts in your life have played out to create a beautiful and complex tapestry, then you are exercising your crown chakra. The goal is to be able to develop it to the point that you can see even beyond your own experience into the rest of the universe.

For instance, suppose you happen across an auto accident. You are the third or fourth car in the area. In other words, everybody else sees the accident. Yet, you are the only one to act. You hop out of your car and rush to the scene to check on the victims. You dial the authorities on the way, to bring in help. Why? How many things had to play out exactly as they did for you to be there at that time, and be the one to help?

Heroic actions are a consequence of your chakras being clear and free. Having a highly developed crown chakra is the final step of that, and is the first step to truly heroic and memorable action. Heroism isn't just doing big things. Heroism is doing the right things over and over again, and improving the lives of all those you meet.

Conclusion

We have covered a lot of ground in this first chapter. We have learned that our psychological wellbeing is a consequence of our energetic balance in the energy centers of our body, called the chakras. There are many of them throughout the body, and each location is associated with a function. Clearing out the chakras will help amplify their function and result in a greater quality of life. The goal is to have all of the chakras working in harmony, so you can be a living manifestation of a higher purpose.

In the next chapters, we will explore some ways of making this a reality. I will show you how to awaken and clean out the chakras. Don't take this lightly, please. It is a journey and one that will take many years to complete. As you will find out, however, the results are well worth the patience and persistence.

Chapter 2
Connection between the Aura and the Chakras

Energy is not constrained to lie within our bodies. In fact, the energy can spill out into the universe. In particular, each and every one of us has a sort of "force field" that is a halo of energy surrounding our bodies. This is called the aura.

The aura is related to the chakras in that it is a manifestation of universal energy. While the chakras are anchored within the body and relate more to our overall position in life, the aura is a reflection of our temporary energetic state. It's a sort of "mood ring" that indicates how we are feeling at any given time. We'll get into the colors of the aura in a minute, but first let's consider how this energetic field interacts with other sources of energy.

We would be mistaken to think that our energy exists in isolation of all other beings. Nothing could be farther from the truth. The fact is that our aura interacts with that of the people around us, and we aren't even aware of it. There is ample evidence to demonstrate this, and we've all experienced it at one time or another in our lives.

If you have felt anxious in a room full of people, then this is a consequence of the interaction of so many auras. Some people are better able to deal with these interactions than others, and for those who aren't as adept the result is what can be called social anxiety. Really, it's just a consequence of the interference pattern of so many auras in one time and place.

One particularly uncanny manifestation is the phenomenon of knowing when you are being watched. If you've felt like you have eyes in the back of your head that let you know when someone is burning a hole in your head, then this is a consequence of the interaction of your aura. This was particularly useful for our ancestors, who had to worry about warring with neighboring tribes. If you didn't know you were being stalked, you were in trouble. Of course, in modern times this isn't so much a concern, but the ability persists nonetheless.

Another example is the calming effect certain people can have on us. This is most startling when it is experienced in the presence of a stranger. Sure, the effect can be written off when it is experienced in the context of the visit of an old friend, but such a rational explanation is lacking when we are meeting someone new. A sensation of calm when meeting a stranger is a consequence of the interconnectedness of our species, rather than some feeling of familiarity.

On the other hand, some individuals can influence us to feel outright agitated and irritable. This is, once again, a consequence of aural interactions. Some people do not have compatible auras, at least at a given moment in time, and this can result in a feeling of anxiety and irritability in the part of one or both individuals. This can happen in the absence of any verbal of physical cue, since it doesn't rely on normal communication.

Similar to this is the sensation of being drained in the presence of another person. When you feel your vital energy is being drained around someone else, this can be a consequence of many things. They could simply be upset, having a bad day, or particularly sad. In some cases, the individual may even be a sort of psychic vampire. Yes, there are people out there that feed on the energy of others. Of course, they don't drink blood in the literal sense, but their consumption of our vital energy is no less dangerous. Such individuals should be avoided, as our precious life force is not in infinite supply, and should be looked after with great care.

More usefully, some people have a great gift for unconsciously reading the auras of others. This manifests itself as an acute sense of empathy and ability to read others. While some may chalk it up to the ability to read subtle body language, it is more likely a consequence of an individual having an especially sensitive aura of their own that reacts to the energetic fluctuations of another person. If you've ever known that someone wasn't being truthful when they said they were OK, then this may have been happening to you. Or you could also be Sherlock Holmes!

While we have focused on our aural experiences with respect to other human beings, it does not end there. All living beings possess an aura, and this means even animals have one. Dogs and humans are particularly well adapted to be sensitive to each other's auras, due to our long-standing symbiotic relationship. Other living beings are included in this. Plants, for instance. Yes, it is possible to have an aural connection to something as simple as a cactus. While it may not be as dynamic as our connection to man's best friend, it exists nevertheless.

You may be wondering if this extends to physical structures. The answer would be "yes". Since we know from centuries of physical inquiry that energy is a conserved quantity (meaning it can't be created or destroyed, only change forms), when there is activity in a location there can be a record of it. This results in locations having a certain vibe, even when there is nobody else around. If you've ever visited an old home and been creeped out, then you've certainly experienced this.

Aural Colors and their Meanings

Green: Green is a color that indicates harmony and balance. It is a reflection of personal development and growth, empathy and a desire to change and transform. Darker shades of green can indicate possessiveness or a persistent fear of being unworthy of love.

Blue: Blue indicates orderliness, peace and the ability to speak the truth. It is indicative of calm and a state of being serious. If a person has a predominantly blue aura, it can be surmised that they have a powerful sense of their purpose in life.

Purple: This reflects an integration of both the spiritual and the physical realm. This is coupled with intuition and a powerful imagination. These lucky individuals may be capable of lucid dreaming or astral travel.

Gold: Gold indicates connection to the higher power, the universal life energy. This is typical of devoutly religious people who aren't merely putting on a show. The presence of a gold aura indicates a state of high spiritual development.

Pink: Pink suggests softness with a strong sense of love for others. It is the color of compassion and kindness; a consequence of a gentle nature. Darker shades could indicate the person gives too much of themselves to others.

Red: Red is the color of our most basic primal urges. It shows a connection to our base self and the Earth. Those with a red aura are lovers of life. Dark shades are indicative of anger deeply seated within the psyche.

Orange: Orange is associated with creativity and ambition. Those with an orange aura are emotionally expressive.

Black: While this is typically associated with negativity, it can actually mean the person is peaceful.

Grey: Grey aura indicates the individual is undergoing a sort of spiritual awakening.

Aural Cleansing

Since our energy field interacts with the world around us on a continual basis, we may often want to cleanse it of unwanted influences. One major method is the chakra meditation I will teach you in a later chapter, however, there are other, less involved ways to deal with this issue.

Since our aura interacts with nature, one great way to cleanse it is to interact with the Earth on a regular basis. This is as simple as going for a stroll through a wooded area and being present in the moment. Try to disable your cell phone and get far away from other electromagnetic influences when you do this. Take the time to really unplug for a while. Practice deep breathing by using your diaphragm to draw in the healing and cleansing energy of mother Earth.

If you want to take it a step further, you can try something like:

- Tree hugging – it's not just for hippies. Close your eyes and attune yourself to the aura of the tree, allowing it to integrate with your own.

- Walk barefoot in nature to solidify your connection to the Earth.

- Practice some mindfulness meditation under a tree. This can also be done with the meditation I will teach you in a later chapter.

Chapter 3
Chakra Balancing

We've already discussed how the imbalance of energy in your chakras results in negative consequences in your day to day life. The process of fixing this imbalance is called··· Chakra balancing. How original, right? So what exactly is this balancing act?

One thing to keep in mind is that none of these chakras exist in isolation. It's not as if we only have a root or sacral chakra. Rather, there is a collection of chakras and they work together as a system. When thinking about chakra balance, you should consider the interconnected nature of their existence. Imbalances can often have a ripple effect. For instance, an imbalance in the root chakra that results from a lack of basic necessities is going to cause issues in the sacral chakra, and result in problems with your emotional wellbeing. This results in issues with emotional intimacy, and your overall sense of self. Your judgement becomes clouded and you can't see the forest for the trees. It is only by identifying the root cause of all of this that you can take corrective action. This requires thinking in terms of your chakras as a system.

Aside from dealing with catastrophic incidents, the necessity of chakra balancing extends into everyday stress and anxiety. Modern society is stressful, and this results in energetic imbalances. One obvious manifestation of this are feelings of being overwhelmed, of stress, of anxiety. These sensations are prevalent here in the West, even to the extent that it is thought to be normal. In some circumstances our state of stress and anxiety is even seen as a badge of honor. It is a sort of proof that we are working hard and being productive. The reality is that stress and anxiety hamper productivity and diminish quality of life. There is therefore a pressing need to practice chakra balancing even if you are otherwise OK and not in an overly distressed state.

By balancing the flow of energy into and out of your chakras, you will improve your ability to deal with the everyday stresses we all experience. Needless to say, this improves quality of life immensely. In a later chapter we' ll go into the how, but first let' s take an overview of some of the methods that are known to bring the chakras into balance

- Pranayama (breath work)

- Yoga, or other exercise focused on the mind-body connection

- Energetic healing (reiki)

- Meditation

We are going to focus on meditation and self-inquiry as the route to chakra balancing, as it is one of the most effective that you can practice on your own. Meditation will also have many positive effects that carry over into all aspects of life. It is also a great technique to counter-balance the tendency of modern society to diminish our ability to focus.

Though we won't delve into it in this work, yoga and pranayama are great for chakra balance as well as overall health. Even something as simple as breathing is more nuanced than most would expect. In fact, most people simply don't breathe deeply enough. We highly recommend you check out some information on pranayama as it will have health effects that carry over into the rest of your life.

The same can be said of yoga. As we alluded to earlier, we are inundated with stress on a daily basis. Dealing with this in constructive ways is critical. Yoga is a great form of exercise that can be adapted for virtually everyone. It is even appropriate for those that have been relatively sedentary for quite some time. Contrast that to exercise such as running or weightlifting, which requires significant stretching (which yoga also covers!) before you can even safely begin.

Reiki is something less familiar to us in the West. While yoga, breath work, meditation, and chakras are somewhat well known, the practice reiki is relatively obscure. Reiki is actually a word of Japanese origin, meaning "spiritually guided life force energy". The practice of reiki is similar to laying of hands in the Christian religions, whereby energy is channeled into a person for the purposes of healing them. One of the neat aspects of reiki is that it is independent of religion or dogma. It requires no particular spiritual faith to be practiced. If this is something that interests you, there are numerous resources available on the internet to teach you how to practice these techniques.

All of these techniques play a role in chakra balancing and healing. As we said earlier, we will focus on the process of chakra meditation to bring the chakra back into balance.

Chapter 4
An Introduction to Chakra Meditation for Chakra Balance

We have covered what the various chakra are and what they do. We have gained some insight into how critical they are for the functioning of our day to day lives. In the previous chapter we talked a little bit about the various techniques that can be used to bring them into balance. We are going to give you a step by step process for chakra meditation so you can start to bring your chakra into balance.

Begin by sitting in a comfortable position. If you can comfortably cross your legs, that is a fine position to begin with. You want to avoid lying down as this can easily result in falling asleep. While a nap may be helpful, it's not going to help you with your chakra meditation. Keep your spine straight, but not rigid. Comfort is key here. When you are comfortable and upright you want to begin by focusing on each part of your body. Start from your feet and work your way up. Be aware of the sensation in each body part. You want to be aware of any stress, tension, or discomfort. Allow these sensations to melt away as you work your awareness up your body.

Begin to focus on your breath. Don't force your breathing, but you should take deep breaths at a steady pace. You want to practice breathing with your diaphragm. To do this, as you breath gently, push out your abdomen. This will cause your diaphragm to contract and your lungs expand. This lets air deep into your lungs. You will be able to breathe much more deeply than you otherwise would.

While focusing on your breathing, you want to begin to clear your mind. This is extraordinarily difficult, and will take a long time to master. Your mind will begin to wander. This is normal, and expected. You will no doubt think of the day's events, of the things you have to do, of conversations you had. Don't feel anxiety over the fact that your mind is constantly bombarded with thoughts that you can't seem to control. The trick here is to acknowledge the thoughts, as if you are watching them on a screen. Don't allow any emotional response, just sort of let them flow. By focusing on your breathing you will eventually learn to control the parade of thoughts in your head.

It helps to visualize the oxygen you are breathing going into your lungs and into the bloodstream. Picture it on its journey to the rest of your body. Into your muscles and organs. The oxygen is truly the life force of your body. Focus on this for some time.

Next begin to visualize the beating of your heart. Visualize how your body works together as a whole unit. This is a parallel for your chakras. Both your body (the physical) and your chakras (energy) are a system whose parts work together to become more than their sum. Visualize how the breath is the life giving force to all parts of the system.

Once you have this down, you want to visualize that you are inhaling something in addition to the air. Visualize you are breathing in a yellowish orange energy. This energy should fill your entire body and surround it to infuse your aura. Imagine your aura growing stronger and more vibrant with each breath. Spend some time on this step of the process, with the aura growing brighter and larger with each breath. At this point, you are ready to begin focusing on the chakras themselves.

Start by imagining you are infusing the root chakra with energy. It helps to visualize a clockwise vortex of energy that is being fed with each and every breath. In addition to being fed by the energy from your breath, you want to begin drawing energy from the Earth. This energy is the same as from the air, but a different source. You can imagine it as having the same yellowish orange color.

Next start moving up the chakra. Begin energizing the sacral chakra by visualizing the breath and earth infusing it with a clockwise swirling energy. Then start to move your way up your body to the solar plexus, the heart, the throat, third eye, and finally the crown. Spend as much time on each chakra as you feel you need. The important thing is to always start from the bottom (the root chakra) and work your way up. Don' t skip around, even if you feel like one chakra is more important. If that' s the case, simply spend more time on it when its turn has arrived. Remember that the chakra are a system, and you must treat them as such. Don' t skip around!

The last step is to visualize all the chakra at once being fed by the energy from the air and the Earth. Your aura and each chakra should grow in intensity, vibrancy, and clarity with each breath.

Finally, just open up your eyes and relax for a couple of minutes. You may want to practice some awareness around how each part of your body feels. You should feel refreshed and relaxed. This meditation is a stress buster for sure. Try to practice this at least once a day, for 15 to 30 minutes.

So to recap, here's a synopsis of the process

1. Sit in a comfortable position with your spine straight but not rigid. Practice awareness of your whole body starting from your feet.

2. Focus on your breath and try to dismiss your thoughts as your mind races. Practice deep breathing.

3. Visualize the beating of your heart. Practice awareness of your body as a system and how your breath feeds the whole thing.

4. Imagine you are breathing in a life-giving energy with each breath. The energy is yellowish orange. It wraps your body and charges your aura.

5. Visualize this energy charging your root chakra. You want to also start bringing energy from the Earth. These energies rotate clockwise and grow in intensity and vibrancy.

6. Start moving up to the sacral chakra, and the rest of the chakras in turn. Don' t skip around, but feel free to spend as much or as little time at each one as you need.

7. Then imagine all the chakras being charged by your breath and Earth simultaneously. They should all grow in intensity and clarity with each breath.

8. Finally open your eyes and sit quietly for a couple of minutes. Practice mindfulness around your whole body and observe how great it feels.

That's "all there is to it", so to speak. While this seems simple in theory, you will find that it takes quite a bit of practice to master. In particular, the process of focusing on your breathing and dismissing your other thoughts is quite difficult. I would advise spending quite a bit of time at this step with each meditation.

The key here is going to be patience and perseverance. You will have to do this every day, for quite some time. It will get easier as time progresses, and you will begin to see more pronounced effects. You will be more relaxed, focused, and have a greater overall sense of wellbeing than you did before. The benefits of this meditation are quite enormous if done properly, so please stick with it even if it is difficult at first.

A word about responsibility, though. Many people will claim they don' t have time for this. That' s just a lie we tell ourselves. We certainly have time. How much time do we spend watching T.V. or watching YouTube videos? Virtually everyone can spare 15-30 minutes a day for meditation. As a matter of fact, some of the most successful people in the world practice meditation. If someone running two businesses and raising a family has time to meditate daily, so do you!

Conclusion

Thank you again for taking time to read this book!

I hope this book was able to help you to gain a deeper understanding and appreciation of the interconnectedness of our universal energy. This energy manifests itself in our auras, which are a reflection of our current mood and mental state. Aural interactions are responsible for our ability to experience emotions just by our proximity to another person, or location. This happens due to interference between multiple auras.

Our more innate energy resides in the chakras. Like the other systems in the body, the chakra must be in balance for our physical and mental health to be at their peak levels. Regular chakra meditation can help to keep energetic imbalances in check and keep your physical and mental health strong.

The next step is to persist in chakra meditation on a daily basis. Consistent practice will help you on multiple levels. It's certainly not easy, but with time it will become more so.

If you have enjoyed this book, please be sure to leave a review and a comment to let us know how we are doing so we can continue to bring you quality eBooks.

Thank you and good luck!

Kundalini

The Kundalini Awakening Guide for Healing and Unlocking Your Spiritual Power

Disclaimer

purchaser or reader of these materials. Any perceived slight of any individual or organization is purely unintentional.

Table of Contents

Introduction

I want to thank you and commend you for taking the time to read the book, "Kundalini: The Kundalini Awakening Guide for Healing and Unlocking Your Spiritual Power."

This book aims to deliver an understanding of what Kundalini practice is, plus a brief history and other background information to help you gain a more complete context. This book also includes suggestions on how to start your Kundalini practice in order to heal and empower your body, mind, and spirit.

We will begin our investigation of Kundalini by describing the spirit's connection to the body. We will follow this with a brief tour of prehistory and history to gain a better understand of the roots of Kundalini practice. Next, we will delve into the concepts of spiritual awakening.

In the next chapter, we will look at healing the body and how Kundalini practice makes the body's own natural ability to heal itself more effective. Along the way, we'll take a glimpse at the dangers of recreational drugs, especially when mixing them with Kundalini practice, plus some of the more positive practices which are compatible with Kundalini yoga. Then, in chapter 5, we'll address the topic of spiritual power, discussing some of the potential dangers and how they are overcome. In chapter 6, we focus on chakras, nadis, and the subtle body to understand where our Kundalini practice will be focused. And finally, we will look at an overview of the Kundalini awakening practice itself, acquainting us with some of the masters of the past, and gaining a greater insight into the details of Kundalini practice.

Though the thousands of details of Kundalini practice are beyond the scope of this book, these chapters give you a broad understanding of what is involved in awakening Kundalini energy. When you have finished reading, you will have a clear idea of the challenges and the benefits of Kundalini awakening.

Thanks again for taking the time to read this book, I hope you enjoy it!

Chapter 1: The Spirit's Connection to the Body

What is Kundalini? According to yogi and mystic, Sadhguru, "The word 'kundalini' generally refers to that dimension of energy that is yet to realize its potential. There is a huge volume of energy within you that is yet to find its potential." Kundalini comes from the Sanskrit word which means "coiled one," like a snake or a rope. Masters of the Kundalini yoga practice characterize this energy as residing at the base of the spine, coiled like a snake and summoned to rise through the chakras (points within the body) to the crown chakra at the top of the head.

Until 1969, Kundalini yoga had been kept from the world at large. Yogi Bhajan, realizing that the world was undergoing dramatic changes, decided to release the secrets of Kundalini yoga to humanity so that we could all be better prepared for the transition facing us.

For those of us who know we are spiritual beings in possession of physical, but temporary, bodies, we are sometimes made aware of this connection between body and spirit.

And how is the spirit connected to the animal body? This has been the subject of great philosophical discussion throughout the ages. In Kundalini, we look at points, called chakras, within the physical body, which are like portals to parts of something called the subtle body. These seem to act as a switchboard between spirit and body, linking the two.

In the spiritual realm, there is no space or objects, so the positions of these chakras reside in the physical realm, but

1

they each represent different characteristics of the unconscious, spiritual self. Through Kundalini practice, the spiritual self is awakened.

Each teacher has their own way of describing the meaning or essence of Kundalini. There are many approaches. This book will touch on some of those unique practices, but will concentrate on the most common elements of Kundalini practice.

The Hidden Treasure

There is a story of a friendless beggar which epitomizes the potential of Kundalini Yoga.

Once upon a time, a lonely beggar, who had always lived in terrible poverty, sat under a tree asking for alms from passersby. He survived on the few coins people threw his way. After a long life existing this way, he died. His body remained under the tree. Without friends or relatives, no one cared to remove his body for a proper burial. So, the people who lived nearby decided to bury him where he had lived—under the tree.

After digging for a little while, the people encountered a chest filled with great treasure.

Within a few feet of the lonesome beggar sat a chest full of gold, and the fool had been sitting on top of it his entire life, begging. If only he had taken the time to dig down within his chosen spot, he could have been a very wealthy man.

In a way, the beggar represents those who do not practice Kundalini. They remain poor in spirit and yet they are so close to a veritable gold mine of treasure. The practice of Kundalini allows us to dig down to find the hidden treasure within us.

How was the beggar to know that underneath him was a good place to dig? It all has to do with awareness of one's surroundings. If we never look, we will never find. If we open our consciousness and wonder what might be there, then we are primed to discover great wonders we never could have otherwise imagined.

Welcome to the journey of Kundalini yoga practice.

Chapter 2: Borne Out of Ancient Teachings

The Dark Mists of Prehistory

The story of humanity before records were first written remains hidden from our view, but we have clues to a great many things happening beyond that veil which resides at the edge of history. Amongst the threads of ancient history and human prehistory, the philosophical building blocks which ultimately became Kundalini practice were laid down. Here, we will attempt to piece together some of those threads to get a sense of where this wisdom may have originated.

The earliest glimpse remains only a tangential clue, at best. It comes from a Greek philosopher named Plato (c.427–c348 BC). In his dialogues, *Timaeus* and *Critias* (the latter of the two remains unfinished), he told of a remarkable island empire named Atlantis. Mention this name to most any scientist these days and you're likely to receive a cold glare of disdain. To most professionals, "Atlantis" is a blasphemous name worthy of scorn. Ironically, their disdain for the subject left the field wide open for other researchers. Scientist and writer, Rod Martin Jr., found evidence of an Atlantis-like event occurring right when Plato said the legendary island empire succumbed to the sea. Three separate pieces of scientific evidence, each from a different discipline, coincide with that controversial date—Plato's approximation of 9600 BC.

In the science of oceanography, we find evidence of sea level rising for thousands of years after the depths of the last glacial period of the current Ice Age. Then, at 9620 BC, there seems to have been a sudden, 2-meter drop in sea level, consistent with an Atlantis-sized piece of land collapsing somewhere in the oceans of Earth.

In the science of glaciology, we find evidence of a major volcanic eruption in the Greenland ice core at GISP2, for 9620.77 BC.

And, in the science of paleoclimate, we find evidence from a number of proxies for the sudden end to the Younger Dryas Big Freeze, 9620 BC.

Though these don't directly prove Atlantis existed, each of these directly support the notion that a large body of land in the Atlantic subsided on Plato's legendary date.

The refugees of Atlantis, if that land really did exist, would have taken with them a far more ancient culture and technology into a primitive Ice Age world now known as Eurasia.

Could some other myths be related to the children of Atlantis? Could the wisdom of India have been influenced as those children migrated across Eurasia, starting 6,000 years before our own history began?

The Bhagavad Gita

Traditionalists claim that the Gita was written in the third or fourth millennium BC, about at the end of the Dvapara Yuga—the third age, which was supposed to have lasted 864,000 years, and, supposedly, ended about the time the Gita was delivered—nominally 3139 BC. This was during the earliest days of our own history. According to that reasoning, we are currently living in the Kali Yuga (432,000 years)—the age of the demon named "Kali"—the age of vice, strife, discord, quarrel, and contention.

The Gita tells of a pause in the Kali Yuga—a 10,000-year Golden Age. Could the renewed interest in spirituality in our modern times be the leading edge of this Golden Age? If so, then Kundalini yoga is playing its part in establishing a period of greater health, love and spirituality amidst the Age of Strife.

The Vedas and Hinduism

The word "véda," in Sanskrit, means knowledge or wisdom.

There are four key bodies of philosophical work in Hinduism, besides the Bhagavad Gita. These are:

- Rigveda,

- Yajurveda,

- Samaveda, and

- Atharvaveda.

Each of these main Vedic texts are divided into subcategories:

Samhitas (benedictions and mantras)

Aranyakas (ceremonies, rituals, sacrifices, and symbolic gestures)

Brahmanas (commentaries)

Upanishads (discussing meditation, spiritual knowledge, and philosophy)

The Rigveda is said to have been composed between about 1700–1100 BC. This period saw the time of Moses, the Minoan civilization destroyed partly by the massive eruption of Thera (erroneously thought to have been Atlantis by some), and the rise of the Mycenaean civilization of Agamemnon and the Trojan War. It also saw the Phoenicians develop writing, the legends of Jason and his Argonauts, Medea and her golden dragon, and the Phoenicians first building a port at what is today Lisbon, Portugal.

Each of the Vedic books was a compilation from numerous sources. Yajurveda and Atharvaveda are thought to have been compiled between about 1200–1000 BC. Some parts of Samaveda were thought to have been created during the early Rigveda period, but were likely brought together in its final form about the same time that the Yajurveda and Atharvaveda were compiled.

The following description is supposedly from one of the minor Vedic texts called Samarangana Sutradhara and describes what was termed to have been a "true" story, rather than a parable or metaphor.

"Inside the circular air frame, place the mercury-engine with its electric/ultrasonic mercury boiler at the bottom center. By means of the power latent in the mercury which sets the driving whirlwind in motion, a man sitting inside may travel a great distance in the sky in a most marvelous manner. Four strong mercury containers must be built into the interior structure. When those have been heated by controlled fire from iron containers, the vimana develops thunder-power through the mercury. At once it becomes like a pearl in the sky."

If such a device ever existed, it has left traces only in the myths of the world. Consulting a Sanskrit-English dictionary, *vimana* was found to mean a spired or conical roof as on a temple or shrine, like the Taj Mahal. Perhaps the shape alone was not sufficient for the flight characteristics of this device. Could it be that vimanas of ages past were only made of certain materials which contributed to the effect? We may never know for sure. Could such technology have been related to the children of Atlantis? Much more research will be required to find possible answers.

Hinduism itself is a mixture of many cultural philosophies with some shared beliefs and many unique, localized beliefs not held in common by the whole. After Christianity (2.2 billion), and Islam (1.6 billion), Hinduism (1.1 billion) is the third largest religion by number of followers.

Two other key religions have been borne out of Hinduism—Buddhism and Sikhism. There are a great many things these three share in common, but also a great many differences. Kundalini yoga comes to us through Hinduism and Sikhism.

Hinduism and Yoga

Many scholars speculate that yoga techniques originated about the fifth or sixth centuries BC. Yoga teachings can be found in Hinduism, Buddhism and Jainism. The four yoga systems are Mantra yoga, Hatha yoga, Laya yoga and Rāja yoga, but there is a broad array of practices, schools, and goals among the yogic disciplines. The Shiva Samhita text states that Kundalini awakening can be achieved by any one of the four yogas, though today, Kundalini yoga is considered by many to be equivalent to Laya yoga. Some of the earliest written records of yoga teachings come from the Hindu Upanishads.

Sikhism

After Buddhism (488–535 million), Taoism (12–173 million), and Shinto (100 million), Sikhism is the 7th largest religion at 28 million members worldwide, just ahead of Judaism (14 million).

Long after the Mongol Empire of Genghis Khan had crumbled, Muslim hordes invaded the Indian subcontinent and established the Mughal Empire (1526–1857). This new ruling class were Turco-Mongols from Central Asia. Like the modern Turks, their religion was Islam. Monotheistic Sikhism was developed shortly before the early Mughal reign, from the teachings of Guru Nanak (1469–1539), said to be the First Guru of the religion.

Nanak had been recognized early on as a very spiritual young boy and received training to cultivate his natural talents. At age 30—about 1499 AD, seven years after Christopher Columbus set off on his first voyage of discovery—Nanak had a vision which interrupted his planned spiritual training.

When he did not return home for several days, people thought he had drowned. Yet, when he finally did return, he had strong words for the townspeople. "There is neither Hindu nor Mussulman (Muslim), but only man. So whose path shall I follow? I shall follow God's path. God is neither Hindu nor Mussulman and the path which I follow is God's."

This pronouncement marked the beginning of Sikhism.

From the history of the period, it seems that the Muslim conquerors were intolerant of other religions. When Guru Arjan and Guru Tegh Bahadur, two Sikh gurus, refused to convert to Islam, they were brutally tortured and then murdered by their Muslim rulers. This prompted a call for religious freedom which Sikhism, and others, eventually received.

Sikh men wear turbans on their heads and are frequently confused with Arabs or Muslims. Tragically, right after 9/11, one American young man murdered a Sikh service station owner in Phoenix, Arizona, in retribution for the attack blamed on Muslims. Because the Sikh had worn a turban, the young man thought he was Muslim. This remains a common misconception.

Kundalini Yoga

The Yoga-Kundalini Upanishad is a part of the Muktika canon originating from some time before 1656 AD.

Swami Nigamananda (1880–1935) insisted that his own brand of Kundalini (Laya) yoga was not part of Hatha yoga, though some had claimed a relationship between the two forms of yoga. In 1935, Hindu Swami Sivananda (1887–1963) wrote his own book on Kundalini Yoga.

In 1968, Sikh Yogi Bhajan (born Harbhajan Singh Puri; 1929–2004), began promoting a form of Kundalini Yoga he had developed. The Sikh established the 3HO teaching group (Healthy, Happy, Holy Organization). Though none of the Sikh gurus had ever taught yoga, and even though the key Sikh holy book, *Guru Granth,* had refuted the yoga practice, Yogi Bhajan's followers insist that his form of Kundalini Yoga is based on Sikh Dharma principles.

Some Sikh's, like Dr. Trilochan Singh, have strongly criticized Bhajan's work. He called it "a sacrilegious hodgepodge," and unSikh-like. Yet today, many followers of Bhajan's teachings hold great reverence for his wisdom and for the benefits they have derived from that wisdom. As with any subject, a teaching is only as good as far as it produces clearly defined results.

In the next chapter, we will delve into how Kundalini yoga can help you achieve spiritual awakening.

Chapter 3: Awakening

Kundalini yoga teachings have been influenced by Shaktism (Hindu worship of the Mother Goddess, Shakti), and Tantrism (Hindu practice of channeling universal or divine energy into the human level of existence).

Awakening of the Kundalini energy is accomplished through regular performance of meditation, chanting mantra, pranayama (control over breath or life force), and yoga asana (sitting in a firm but relaxed position).

For example, in pranayama, breath is controlled and even altered in order to achieve different, specific results within the body. Such conscious control puts the Kundalini yoga practitioner in greater awareness of the body and its feelings.

We liken this increased awareness to that of a person shining a light on places which had, until now, remained dark.

Yoga Sutras of Patanjali

Hindu sage, Patanjali, around 400 AD, wrote his own Yoga Sutras. In them, he discussed certain breathing techniques which are used before concentration meditation. His Samadhi Padi Sutra describes being absorbed in spirit. His Sadhana Pada Sutra talks of being immersed in spirit. His Vibhuti Pada Sutra tells how one can achieve supernatural abilities and gifts. And his Kaivalya Pada Sutra discusses absolute freedom.

Pranayama Techniques

Some of the spiritual breathing techniques include: ·

1. Agni-prasana ("breath of fire").

2. Agnisar pranayama (breathing from the abdomen).

3. Anuloma pranayama (an alternate form of nostril breath).

4. Bhastrika pranayama (diaphragmatic breathing which drive fast, forceful inhales and exhales). This is used to clear the nadis (subtle body channels).

5. Bhramari pranayama (a humming while breathing, sounding like a bee).

6. Kumbhaka pranayama (retaining breath on both inhale and exhale).

7. Pratiloma pranayama (another technique for cleansing the nadis or subtle body channels and awakening the Kundalini energy by alternating the inhale between left and right nostrils; exhale from both nostrils).

8. Shtali pranayama (breath is taken in over an extended tongue, curled up at the end, yielding a cooling effect).

Kundalini Yoga Practice

Part of the purpose of Kundalini practice is to raise your own level of awareness of your entire body. This is meant to prepare the body and its nervous system (especially the brain) to handle the energy emitted when the Kundalini rises along the nadis (channels or pathways) through the chakras (nodes within the subtle body).

Each action taken—or kriya—renders a specific result in the awakening of the Kundalini energy. Some results can seem quite pleasant. Others can be somewhat uncomfortable.

Among its many benefits, Kundalini yoga is said to free us from our karma and to help us gain an understanding of our life's purpose (dharma).

According to Yogi Bhajan, "Kundalini Yoga consists of active and passive asana-based kriyas, pranayama, and meditations which target the whole body system (nervous system, glands, mental faculties, chakras) to develop awareness, consciousness and spiritual strength."

Degrees of Awakening

One spiritual student described several levels of spiritual awakening he had achieved on his journey. In his own experience, the first was a faint awareness of self as distinct and separate from others. Next was a robust and profound awareness of the source of awareness within the self—behind the ego self. This, he characterized as equivalent to looking into a spiritual mirror. After this, he found an awareness of a true self connected to others and distinctly different from the false, separate, ego self. And finally, he described an awakening as not only connected to others, but unconditionally loving; perfectly responsible for the desires, attitudes and actions of others; fearlessly confident; and utterly humble, as if all self-concern had disappeared.

Naturally, each individual will have their own unique experiences as they approach spiritual awakening. But these details help describe the territory you are now entering with your desire to awaken your own Kundalini energy—your own hidden treasure.

Accessing the True Source of Power

We're all familiar with the electric socket. We plug a wire into one and our appliance or light bulb turns on. Yet, the socket is nothing more than an access point. The socket does not create the energy. The true source of the energy is a power station that is likely many miles away.

Adding too many loads to a circuit will draw so much power that it could burn out the connections. If you plug in an air-conditioner, a heater, a toaster, refrigerator, television and computer to one outlet, you will likely blow a fuse. Someone who doesn't realize the dangers might replace the fuse with a copper coin. When their house burns down, they don't understand that the fault was theirs, because they allowed horrendous amounts of energy through the wires of the house and those wires melted, burning down the house as a result

Even a regional power source such as an electrical generating station is limited. It cannot supply infinite power for every possible use.

Our bodies require energy, but as Christ said, man does not live by bread alone. Food only gives the body physical energy. And, like the electrical power station, such nourishment supplies only a limited amount of energy.

In Kundalini practice, you tap into the source of infinite power. Like the circuit fuse, your inability to access all that power all at once protects you from harm. When you learn the proper methods of Kundalini practice, you are preparing your body and subtle body pathways (nadis) for handling more power.

So, be patient with your progress. Enjoy the journey.

Everything you do activates a small part of your Kundalini energy—exercise, rest, involvement in sports and more. In fact, some professional athletes have, at times, plugged into the source of power enough to enter what some call "the zone." This is when everything they do in their game becomes effortless and things magically fall into place with a rhythm and grace few ever experience.

In the next chapter, we will see how Kundalini energy helps to heal the body.

Chapter 4: Healing

The human body heals from proper circulation, proper nutrition, and proper distribution of energy. If you've ever had expert massage after a heavy workout or a stressful day, you understand this idea on a visceral level.

If your body is ever cut, the wound will heal far more quickly when you have proper blood flow to the area of damage. Naturally, a broken blood vessel needs to be repaired first, but when this is taken care of, the area of healing needs to remain fully nourished with food, energy, and oxygen through the blood.

When you use Kundalini yoga techniques, the body's vital pathways are opened for optimum transfer of vital ingredients. In other healing arts, the touch assist has been used to help heal the body once injured or ill. Each spot touched on the surface of the body helps the recuperating person communicate more completely with that part of their body.

Awakening the Kundalini energy is said to generate bio-energetic phenomena which can be felt somatically by the practitioner. This is sometimes called "pranic awakening." Prana can be defined as the essential, life-sustaining energy within the body. Sometimes this pranic awakening is experienced as a vibration. Like a miniature massage, such vibration can open up pathways within the body to help it heal.

Doctors know that if a part of the body remains cold or cool to the touch, even after proper warming, that part of the body is not receiving proper circulation. With one form of communication or another—massage, touch assist, or something else—the natural healing tendency of the body is encouraged to flow on its own.

Kundalini yoga, however, goes much deeper. It touches the very channels of spiritual awareness which connect life-giving spirit to the physical form of the body. When done properly, this can have a profound effect on the body's ability to heal itself.

According to the 3ho.org website of Yogi Bhajan's teachings, "This technology precisely and consciously combines breath, mudra, eye-focus, mantra, body locks, and postures to balance the glandular system, strengthen the nervous system, expand lung capacity, and purify the blood. It brings balance to the body, mind, and soul."

Self-Destruction Through Recreational Drugs

In life, there are many kinds of feeling good. If we're hungry, eating a good meal can supply this. If we're thirsty, a cool drink of clean water can quench our desire.

Feeling high can be achieved in a number of ways. Most of them can be selfish and self-destructive. Recreational drugs are one method which supply a quick, artificial high that disrupts the body's internal pathways and energy. Yogi Bhajan once wrote, "...you are not free by taking drugs. The neurons of the brain will become feeble. You will lose your nostril pituitary sensitivity. You can never smell the subtlety of life. You'll always be dragging your life."

With artificial highs, the individual is left enslaved by the need for their next fix. The selfishness to fulfill that need drives many an addict to do unspeakable crimes.

Any pleasure can become somewhat addictive, but spiritual pleasure tends to disrupt the pattern of selfishness. In order to achieve the extreme pleasure of spiritual awakening which heals the body, a person is confronted with the flawed thinking of separateness. When you connect to Kundalini energy, you find the portal which connects us all. This is a natural high which is far safer than drugs and remains health-affirming rather than health-destructive.

The 3ho.org website adds this warning concerning recreational drug use: "According to yogic thought, drugs interrupt the natural flow of the energy of the chakras and the aura, and put strain on the nervous system to compensate. In addition, the drug-induced high and the powerful energies released from the practice of Kundalini Yoga can get out of control with unpredictable results."

Practices Compatible with Kundalini Yoga

There are, however, many practices which remain compatible with Kundalini yoga and, in fact, bolster the benefits received from Kundalini practice.

In the following sections, we will look briefly at a few of these other practices which are Kundalini "safe."

Yogic Foot Massage for Healing

Kundalini practice develops our ability to "see" into our own body and to the chakras which connect us to the superior realm of spirit at the root of existence.

Yogic foot massage helps us connect with our bodies on a deeply physical level. The light of awareness, through the nerve channels of the body, helps to put us into contact with the various parts of our own body. And this increased awareness leads to greater healing.

Though there are many ways to give a foot massage, the yogic foot massage has the specific objective of stimulating all 72,000 of the nerves which link to the body through our feet.

Using cold water, wash the feet to prepare them. This helps to wake up the nerve endings. For those who use a massage oil, be sure to place a towel underneath the feet. The person doing the massage should prepare their mind. Consider yourself to be in a healing mode. Connect to the divine. If you're uncertain how to connect, simply consider it done. The fearless confidence of certainty is full accomplishment in the realm of spirit. Doubt has no business in such matters.

Feel the prana in your hands, and rub some of the oil, if you use it, between the palms of your hands. Then begin. Please be aware that the proper foot massage will be between ten to fifteen minutes in total, evenly divided between the two feet.

Start with the toes, grabbing each one in turn between your thumb and forefinger, twisting and pulling each segment of the toe. Begin at the base of the large toe and work your way out. After twisting a segment several times, pull up (outward toward the end of the toe) while applying more pressure. Then, move to the next segment toward the tip of the toe—two for the big toe and three for the others—14 phalanges in all.

After the toes, move to the remainder of the foot, massaging in slow, but powerful, circular motions. Use fingers, thumbs, and even your knuckles. Try to cover the entire surface. Start under the base of the big toe and progress toward the base of the little toe. Move down a notch and work your way across to the other side of the foot. With this, you progress down the foot toward the heel.

As a final touch, massage both sides of the ankle's Achilles tendon, ending with a firm but brief squeeze to the tendon and release.

Again, as a reminder, be sure to spend the same amount of time on the second foot. This helps the massage remain balanced.

Sat Nam Rasayan®

Sat Nam Rasayan is a healing technique used on a recipient by someone trained in the art.

Yogi Bhajan once said, "Shuniya means zero. The moment you become zero, then all powers will prevail through you." What does this mean? How can becoming zero give you all power?

Spiritual philosopher and writer Rod Martin Jr. once wrote about an incident which occurred in a first year calculus class in college. The professor had drawn the graph of a function's derivative on the board. The resultant line was equivalent to the X-axis, except for a discontinuity at X = 0, where the value of Y was plus-or-minus infinity. Something about the graph immediately awoke him on a spiritual level. He realized that the graph was also a depiction of the state of ego relative to creation's mechanics. "If X is a measure of ego, and Y is a measure of power over physical reality, then this graph would indicate zero power over the universe at any value of ego other than zero, and infinite power over physical reality at zero ego."

So, the claim mentioned earlier about removing our karma takes on greater significance. Ego is the false self in the physical realm. It is made of physical stuff—action-reaction material—the stuff of dichotomies, like karma.

According to Yogi Bhajan, Sat Nam Rasayan simply means, "Deep Relaxation in the True Identity." The 3ho.org website states, "Entering a state of Sat Nam Rasayan means entering a state of total surrender, becoming nothing, and operating from the state of shuniya. The mind of the Sat Nam Rasayan practitioner becomes transcendent and in the vastness of this consciousness healing can occur."

Bhajan also said, "All he does is put his hand on you. Sometimes he doesn't even touch you. Actually it is the 'Sat Naam' which does the healing. You don't see God working."

Through the meditative mind, which is projected by the practitioner, Sat Nam Rasayan works on a subtle level. This technique permits the healer to contact the five elements within the body (water, earth, air, fire, and ether), as well as the pranic body, and to bring them into balance.

Ayurveda and Using Herbs and Other Healing Foods

Ayurveda is a system of medicine thought to have developed in India during the Vedic period. This system includes general medicine; pediatrics, surgical techniques; treatment of eye, ear, nose, and throat ailments; toxicology; rejuvenation and longevity; aphrodisiacs and fertility; and pacification of spirits possessing the body.

Though Ayurveda has its critics amongst Western practitioners, it must be pointed out that Western medicine has been found repeatedly to be corrupt, fudging records, lying to American Congress, pushing medicines to market long before they could be proven effective or safe, and then paying millions of dollars in damages after making billions in profits off the deaths of, and injuries to, their customers. One Western study did raise a legitimate concern when it found that nearly 21% of Ayurveda patent medicines in America and in India, sold over the internet, contained toxic levels of heavy metals (mercury, lead, and arsenic). I recommend not buying such medicines over the internet, unless you have a laboratory which can test them for toxins.

Along with Ayurveda medicine, good food is an essential ingredient in taking full responsibility for your own body.

Kundalini yoga teachers recommend bitter herbs for improving mental function and awareness sensitivity. They are the remedy for "mental dullness."

In times of stress, they recommend the sweet herbs licorice and *ashwaganda*. These help to stabilize the mind when it is suffering from tumultuous energies.

Arjuna is said to strengthen the heart. *Bala* not only increases libido, but is also a natural anti-inflammatory. *Bala* also promotes good pulmonary function.

It should be obvious that life comes from life. Western medicine's dependence upon petrochemical distillations, far removed from natural substances, seems to be based more on profit motive than upon any concern for health—based upon disease maintenance rather than health maintenance. It's easy to understand how Western medicine became so thoroughly derailed. The Rockefeller family (their fortunes based on monopolizing the petroleum industry) would naturally want other uses for their one product. Thus, we have their tainted investment in medical schools which taught only their type of petrochemical medicine.

Harmony in Gemstones

In much the same way that an electronic "tank" circuit can tune into specific radio frequencies or "stations," various gemstones can tune in to various healing energies.

The 3ho.org website elaborates on the use of gemstones and how to choose a set of stones which are right for you, based on your birthdate.

Your birth day of the month is said to be your Soul number. The number of your month is your Karmic value. The two most significant digits of the year become the Gift number. The entire year gives us the Destiny number. And the full birthdate provides us with the Path number.

In numerology we are always interested in reducing a set of numerals to one digit. In Bhajan's system, this is expanded to include "10" as if it were a single digit. The stones for each number are as follows:

1. Amethyst

2. Ruby

3. Citrine

4. Emerald

5. Aquamarine

6. Lapis

7. Rubellite

8. Topaz

9. Sapphire or Opal

10. Diamond

Let us say that your birthdate is September 23, 1985.

The Soul number would be 2+3 = 5—aquamarine.

The Karma number would be 9 (September)—sapphire or opal.

The Gift number would be 8+5 = 13, 1+3 = 4—emerald.

The Destiny number would be 1+9+8+5 = 23, 2+3 = 5—aquamarine.

The Path number would be 9+2+3+1+9+8+5 = 37, 3+7 = 10—diamond.

Yogi Bhajan recommends the ancient Hebrew system for the most accurate selection of birth stones.

Aries—Sapphire

Taurus—Carnelian

Gemini—Emerald

Cancer—Onyx

Leo—Carnelian

Virgo—Chrysolite

Libra—Tourmaline

Scorpio—Topaz

Sagittarius—Ruby

Capricorn—Garnet

Aquarius—Amethyst

Pisces—Jasper

For stones which focus on powerful healing, Yogi Bhajan recommends lapis, coral, turquoise and carnelian. He indicates that lapis provides great protection and takes sickness away; coral provides balance between negative and positive forces; turquoise draws impurities out of the body; and carnelian helps to purify the blood.

Using this system, we can develop jewellery and prayer beads (malas) which are harmonious to our own unique situation in our current, precious human life.

In the next chapter, we take a look at increasing spiritual power and how Kundalini yoga can help.

Chapter 5: Spiritual Power

Everything comes from spirit. Every physical object, every moment in time, every blade of grass, and every creature has its source in the spiritual realm. The root of existence is spiritual. And like any tree, so long as its roots are healthy, the body of the tree above ground—in the open view of all physical reality—has a chance to survive and thrive.

If spirit is blocked in any way, the body cannot reach its full potential. The mind may suffer, too.

There are many systems for achieving increased spiritual power. But be careful. If you approach the increase of such power with a selfish heart, you risk a great deal of suffering for you and those around you. If, on the other hand, you approach your spiritual empowerment for the benefit of others, then this is no longer a problem.

The Meaning of Selfishness

In Buddhism, selfishness is equated with desire and suffering. It comes from ego which is described as "ignorance." Others have described it as "separateness." Christ talked of the First (egoistic) becoming last (left out in the cold); and the Last (loving and non-self-concerned) becoming first (given the keys to the spiritual kingdom).

Spiritual researcher Rod Martin, Jr. wrote of several experiences testing the boundaries of selfishness and ego. In one instance—an evening in 1971—while undergoing spiritual counseling, he found that he had given up ego entirely for a few, brief seconds, after having been asked to consider giving to others without any thought of return.

One moment, he was sitting in a chair facing his spiritual counselor; the next, he was 15 feet above the ground, and 12 feet off of his body's left shoulder. From this position, he could see everything around him, including the closed window blinds between him and his body. He did not feel comfortable looking in all directions at once (360° spherical vision), but he could see clearly everything around him, though he had no physical eyes with which to see. These few, precious moments were filled with a lack of spiritual blindness, all because he had found a crack in ego and had escaped from it for those few moments.

In another incident, which Martin describes in detail in his book, *The Art of Forgiveness*, he suffered six different assaults in rush-hour traffic. All of those assaults were rude and selfish at best. Some of them were downright dangerous. After the sixth such assault in as little as two minutes, Martin's rage suddenly turned to bliss and loving forgiveness. He had realized that he had been fully responsible, not only for the feelings of frustration and rage he had created in response to those assaults, but he was also responsible for the assaults themselves. This responsibility was not for anything he had overtly done to them in that present incident. That responsibility was borne out of his spiritual creation of objects toward which he could aim his frustration and rage, and because he had become trapped in selfishness. When he realized his own culpability in the crimes against himself, the knowledge of this truth suddenly set him free—far freer than he has ever been, before or since.

At that point, two other miracles occurred. He found it effortless to forgive the six who had assaulted him. In fact, it took him more than thirty years to realize that he had forgotten their crimes against him. His love for them had been that complete. And traffic opened up for him, three lanes of bumper-to-bumper traffic suddenly and impossibly becoming two. For four minutes, he traversed that gauntlet—an empty center lane for two miles ahead, and two walls of snarling traffic, one on either side.

When you awaken Kundalini energy, if you remain blinded by selfishness, you cannot accurately control the energy for the purposes of righteous good. This could be compared to looking into a nuclear furnace without wearing protective gear. This is why taking the time to get it right at each step is important to your long-term spiritual health.

Spiritual power created the entire physical universe—all several billion galaxies, each with an average hundred billion stars, and several times as many planets. A large percentage of those worlds may contain several trillion life forms each. Such numbers remain rather mind-numbing, but such is the power of spirit.

Be patient and humble as you awaken your own Kundalini energy. Such humility helps to neutralize the blindness of ego.

Developing Spiritual Power

Kundalini rising through the body stimulates the endocrine glands, including the pineal and pituitary glands. Each gland affects certain body functions and the pineal and pituitary are said to affect the body's sensitivity to spiritual awareness.

Ravi Dykema, a Kundalini yoga therapist, stated, "The yogi or yogini who successfully and safely arouses their Kundalini gains a great ally on their spiritual journey. That ally is an energy, a vitality, that smoothes the path, that makes the steep slopes easier to climb, and that acts like a sword to cut through inertia and conditioning." In other words, your own Kundalini energy acts as a supercharged tool in your own spiritual growth.

Potential Dangers

When dealing with powerful energy, there always remains the possibility that something will not go according to plan. Each human body, and each individual's experiences are complex and unique.

The practitioner needs to approach Kundalini arousal with care. On rare occasions, Kundalini energy can be activated prematurely, causing disruptive energy within the body, including insomnia, panic attacks, twitching, shaking, arm waving, psychic phenomena, and even a sense of being overwhelmed.

Such disruptive arousal of Kundalini energy is rare, but it's better to be aware of these things before beginning. Some people are more sensitive to the power of chanting mantras or sitting in the presence of an influential spiritual teacher. Ecstatic religious experiences, sexual orgasms, and psychotropic drugs can also trigger disruptive Kundalini energy.

The key problem is that your bodily system has not yet become mature before attempting to arouse the Kundalini energy. It must be prepared through proper meditation, chanting and breathing exercises.

If ever this problem arises, the Kundalini practitioner need only return their Kundalini energy to its dormant state. One person found they could do this simply by asserting control over their muscles—a light flexing of the hand or other conscious movement of a body part. Others require the help of a specialist to help them work through a specific set of yoga exercises. Again, such problems are rare.

Taoist Mantak Chia has written at length about this "Kundalini psychosis"—sometimes called "Kundalini syndrome." In his book, *Awaken Healing Light of the Tao,* he provides a technique called "the microcosmic orbit"—a method of grounding the practitioner.

Mantak Chia says that this Kundalini syndrome happens when an overabundance of "hot or Yang Chi" floods up through the body and gets stuck in the brain. The symptoms can last for days, months, or even longer.

A few people have spontaneously triggered Kundalini syndrome even though they had done nothing with energy practices. This is extremely rare. Other accidental Kundalini psychoses have been set off by recreational drug use. This is a form of the drug user's "bad trip."

According to Mantak Chia, a small number of people have activated this Kundalini psychosis because of "doing meditation practices that do not emphasize balanced energy circulation."

In Zen Buddhism, the father of the Japanese Rinzai school, Hakuin Zenji, encountered this phenomenon and called it "Zen illness." He wrote about it in his book, *The Embossed Tea Kettle.* A number of his own students had been afflicted and the malady had nearly killed even him. Ultimately, Hakuin obtained a cure from a Taoist hermit.

In our modern world, some people have been hospitalized, diagnosed as psychotic. Their treatments of psychotherapy and strong medication usually failed, because the modern doctors had no idea about that with which they were dealing.

We have to understand that the root of the problem deals with energy. As said by Mantak Chia, one solution involves moving the energy back down "from the head to the navel or soles of the feet."

The easiest approach involves grounding techniques. Because this Kundalini psychosis comes about from too much "hot" or Yang Chi rushing up to the head, utilizing Yin, or Earth energy, can help move the offending energy downward. Mantak Chia also said that moving Yin upward into the brain can have a cooling effect to neutralize the hot, Yang energy.

How fast is this cure? Many of the symptoms disappear within seconds or minutes. A full cure can take a few days, or possibly as much as three weeks.

Spiritual Benefits

As the Kundalini energy rises through the body, new abilities will sometimes appear to the practitioner. The closer to the top, the more spiritual these abilities become—cosmic consciousness, for instance. The ultimate goal is spiritual liberation, where the individual loses the walls of ego which separate them from the whole.

Chapter 6: Chakras, Nadis and the Subtle Body

Between the physical body and the spiritual self, there resides a subtle body—an arrangement of energies which act as a switchboard between the two realms. At the base of this subtle body, where we would find the coccyx, or base of the spine on the physical, lies the Kundalini energy, coiled and dormant, like a sleeping snake.

The Three Main Nadis

Up through the center of the subtle body run three channels, or nadis. Though there are millions of channels within the body, the three important to Kundalini yoga practices are called ida, pingala, and sushumna.

The ida nadi is known as the "lunar energy" channel, from the Sanskrit word for "comfort," and is given a pale color when represented graphically. This is considered to be a "feminine" form of energy and has a cooling effect on the energies within the subtle body. This travels from the left testicle to the left nostril and is frequently associated with the Ganges river. Ida is also associated with an introverted nature and the right hemisphere of the brain. Ida controls the mental processes. Accessing ida during breathing exercises requires the left nostril to be open.

The pingala nadi is known as the "solar energy" channel, from the Sanskrit word for "tawny"—a warm color, from yellowish brown to orange. This is considered to be a "masculine" form of energy and has a warming effect. This travels from the right testicle to the right nostril and is frequently associated with the Yamuna river. Pingala is also associated with an extroverted nature and the left hemisphere of the brain. Pingala controls the body's vital processes. Accessing pingala during breathing exercises requires the right nostril to be open.

The sushumna nadi connects the base chakra to the crown chakra. Accessing sushumna during breathing exercises requires that both nostrils be open. The way for the Kundalini energy is prepared along all three of the main nadi.

In European lore, the two snakes intertwined around the staff of Hermes (Caduceus of Hermes) has come to symbolize Western medicine, but appears to have roots in the philosophy which gave birth to Kundalini practice.

Major Chakras

Aligned along the center of the subtle body, there are several nodes which connect to various parts of the physical body. The 7 major chakras in the subtle body, from bottom to top, are:

- Muladhara—root chakra

- Svadhishthana—sacral chakra

- Manipura—solar plexus or navel chakra

- Anahata—heart chakra

- Vishuddha—throat chakra

- Ajna—third-eye chakra

- Sahasrara—crown chakra

Kundalini awakening occurs as the energy progresses up along the sushumna nadi from the root chakra—

Muladhara—through all the others toward the crown chakra—Sahasrara.

The three main nadis separate after leaving the Muladhara chakra and proceed up through the subtle body toward the crown chakra, where they meet again.

Minor Chakras

There are said to be 21 minor chakras which are reflected points of the 7 major chakras. For instance, the Hridhiya chakra resides about an inch to the left and an inch down from the Anahata (heart) chakra; and this is where we normally feel our human heartbeat. Some of these are associated with certain body parts—hand, elbow, knee, foot, groin, navel, and others.

Three secret chakras are said to defy detection until the Kundalini energy is fully awakened. These—Golata, Lalata, and Lalana—are said to be located right above the Ajna chakra, not far above the soft palate at the back of the throat.

There are also 7 extra chakras which run down below the Muladhara, associated with parts of the legs.

Atala—hips, governing lust and fear.

Vitala—thighs, governing resentment and anger.

Sutala—knees, governing jealousy.

Talatala—calves, equated to instinctive willfulness and prolonged confusion.

Rasatala—ankles, equated to pure animal nature and the center of selfishness.

Mahatala—feet, equated to an inner blindness and a shrouded realm completely without conscience.

Patala—soles of the feet, equated to the Hindu realm of hell (Naraka), and realm of hatred, torture, malice, and murder.

In the next chapter, we look more deeply into Kundalini practice itself.

Chapter 7: Kundalini Practice

For the safety and most sure-footed progress of the Kundalini yoga practitioner, we recommend that all such practice be supervised by a Kundalini master. Anyone might be able to raise their Kundalini energy all the way to the crown chakra and achieve full, spiritual liberation by themselves. But not everyone is a Yogi Bhajan, or a Siddhartha Gautama Buddha who can achieve Enlightenment on their own. Guidance helps to keep the practitioner on the proper path and away from the dangers of Kundalini psychosis or other pitfalls of selfishness and karma.

Kundalini yoga practice ultimately unburdens or uncovers the Ātman, or inner self, soul, true self. This provides us with a major diversion of Buddhism from the other Hindu-related philosophical viewpoints. Most scholars of Buddhism believe that there is no true self or soul. Yet, at least one spiritual researcher feels that this is not a perfectly accurate portrayal of Buddhism, feeling instead that the avoidance of acknowledging a "true self" is based on the fact that any sense of self is too easily confused with the false, ego self. So, rather than make it harder for Buddhists to give up the source of spiritual ignorance, Buddhist teachers have opted to avoid the entire question of self, preferring for the student to discover the truth upon achieving Enlightenment.

By a combination of breathing exercises, meditation, chants or mantras, and other Kriyas, or "completed actions," the Kundalini practitioner is able gradually to awaken their Kundalini energy, to raise it to the third (navel) chakra, then back down to the root, and finally up through all seven to the crown.

There are many approaches to Kundalini awakening.

- Patañjali's kriya yoga.

- Tantric traditions.

- Hatha traditions, particularly Hatha the Shiva Samhita and Yoga Pradipika.

- Raja yoga.

- Laya yoga.

- Mantra yoga.

- Teachings of Swami Nigamananda.

- Teachings of Swami Sivananda.

- Teachings of Yogi Bhajan.

As we've seen, Kundalini yoga has been influenced by the various parts of its roots in Hinduism, by Buddhism (particularly Zen Buddhism), by Taoism (for example the resolution of Kundalini psychosis), and by Sikhism.

Yogi Bhajan's Approach to Kundalini Awakening

Perhaps one of the most approachable schools of Kundalini awakening is not Hindu, but Sikh, despite the fact that most Sikhs have disavowed yoga as a valid Sikh technique. In the following subsections, the various activities of the Kundalini practitioner are described in greater detail. These will give you a sense of the challenges you will face in moving toward the benefits of Kundalini awakening.

Kriyas

Wait 2–3 hours after eating a light snack before practicing. As with all practice work, make sure cell phones and other distractions are turned off or otherwise blocked from creating a disturbance. Water in a closed container should be readily available for keeping the body hydrated. And natural fiber clothing should be worn instead of synthetics.

Always tune in to the spiritual practice by performing the Adi Mantra before any kriyas, warm-ups, or meditation. This is accomplished by chanting, *"Ong Namo Guru Dev Namo."* three times.

During the actual kriyas, stay alert to what your body is telling you. But also challenge yourself to go a little bit past what you think your limits might be.

For women, avoid strenuous yoga during the heaviest 1–3 days of menstruation. For instance, don't do Breath of Fire, Camel Pose, Bow Pose, Stretch Pose, Root Lock, Locust Pose, Sat Kriya, any inversions, or demanding leg lifts.

After each kriya, drink a good deal of water. Also pay particular attention to your mind, emotions, and physical self. There are more than 40 featured kriyas. Some are simple actions and poses, while others are a more complex series of actions and gestures.

Meditation

Though meditation can be done at any time, it proves to be most beneficial when done at the same time every day. Just before sunrise is particularly good, because it sets the tone for the entire day. In the evening at sunset, or several minutes before going to bed can also prove most favorable.

Of course, be sure to find a place where you will not be disturbed. A natural fiber blanket, cushion, or chair can be used. Regular repetition is far more important than the length of time spent in any one session. For example, 5 minutes of meditation every day is far better than 40 minutes once every week or so.

Before you begin, tune in with the Adi Mantra, then set a clear intention in your mind for the result of your meditation. This initiating intention helps to set the direction of your meditation. This acts as sort of a homing beacon which helps guide your spirit through the period of meditation, much as instruments on an airplane guide the craft toward its physical destination.

There are nearly a hundred featured meditation routines. Like the kriyas, some are simple and some are more complex.

Pranayama (Breathing)

By adjusting the type of breathing and your breathing rate, you can alter your state of mind. Yogi Bhajan recommends three different rates:

- 8 breaths per minute

- 4 breaths per minute

- 1 breath per minute

Not every breathing routine is amenable to these breathing rates. For instance, Breath of Fire requires a rapid, rhythmic, and continuous sequence of breaths.

The recommended breathing routines include:

- Long deep breathing

- Alternate nostril breathing

- Breath of fire

- Suspending the breath

- Segmented breath

- Sitali breath

- Cannon breath

- Whistle breath

- Lion breath

- Sitkari breath

- Vatskar breath

Mudra

The mudra practice involves various positions of the hands, which act as energy maps of health and consciousness. Each special combination of positions, curling, crossing, and stretching of fingers, thumbs, and full form of the hand, is associated with a different aspect of the body-energy system.

The key mudras used in Kundalini awakening are,

- Ravi or Surya Mudra—Seal of Sun, Life.

- Shuni Mudra—Seal of Patience.

- Gyan Mudra—Seal of Knowledge.

- Buddhi Mudra—Seal of Mental Clarity.

- Venus Lock.

- Pranam Mudra—Prayer Pose.

For example, the Gyan Mudra requires that the practitioner touch the index finger tip and the thumb tip together, while the other three fingers remain straight.

Other Practices

Asanas are postures in which the practitioner places their body in order to direct the body's energy flows. Each asana can be used as an exercise, a meditation, a connection to energy flow, and even as a diagnostic tool.

Eye focus can be an essential part of meditations or kriyas, training the eyes on a specific location like the third-eye point, tip of the nose, tip of the chin, or top of the head.

Bandhas are also called "body locks," and are basically positions held and light pressures maintained in order to affect posture, energy flow, and in contacting the Kundalini energy in order to gently coax it to rise.

Sadhana is a form of committed prayer that gives your life direction and purpose.

Conclusion

Thank you again for taking the time to read this book!

I hope this book was able to help you to understand the scope of commitment required of you in pursuing Kundalini awakening. Also, I hope you appreciate the boundless joy that awaits you upon your completion of your Kundalini practice.

The next step is to contact a Kundalini master near you for lessons and guidance.

If you have enjoyed this book, please be sure to leave a review and a comment to let us know how we're doing so we can continue to bring you quality ebooks.

Thank you and good luck!

Preview of: Meditation: How to Relieve Stress by Connecting Your Body, Mind and Soul

Introduction

Thank you for taking the time to read the book, *"Meditation: How to Relieve Stress by Connecting Your Body, Mind and Soul"*.

In this day and age, it's not easy to keep your sanity in check. With all the work you have to do, and everything else you have to handle, sometimes, your mind really suffers. And when that happens, it'll be hard for you to continue with what you're doing.

However, it doesn't mean there's no answer to your problems anymore. With the help of this book, you'd learn various meditation techniques that could take your stress away, and help you get connected to your mind, body, and soul!

When you get in tune with your mind, body, and soul, it will be easier for you to understand what's going on with your life, and in your world. And with that, you can be a better, more productive person—and that's exactly the kind of person you'd like to be!

Keep reading this book now to find out how!

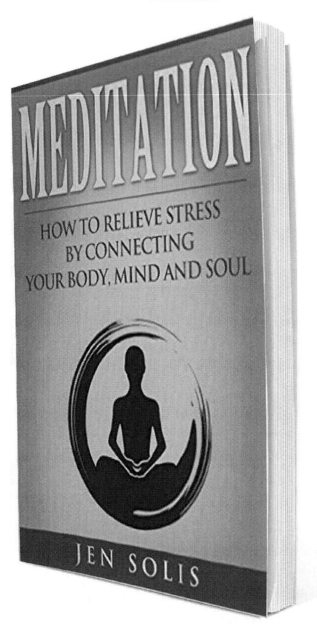

Search on amazon to check out this book.

Check out my book on Mindfulness!

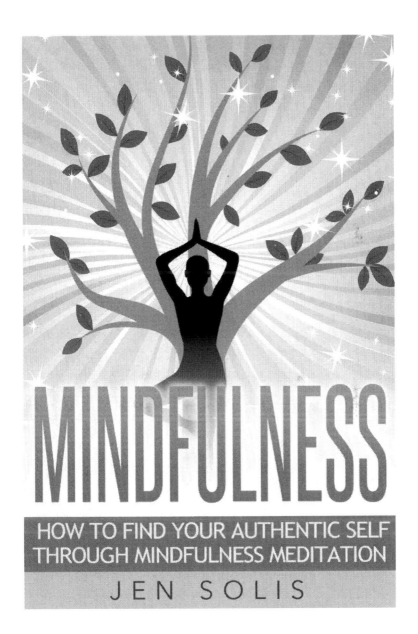

Go to Amazon's book page for "Mindfulness: How to Find Your Authentic Self through Mindfulness Meditation"

Check out my author page for more books that you might be interested in!

Click here to visit my author page on amazon.com.

Some of the books you'll find there are:

YOGA: Essential Yoga Poses for Taking Control Over Your Mind

Meditation: How to Find Inner Peace and Relieve Stress and Anxiety

Meditation: How to Relieve Stress by Connecting Your Body, Mind and Soul

Mindfulness: How to Find Your Authentic Self through Mindfulness Meditation

Zen: How to Practice Zen Everywhere in Your Daily Life

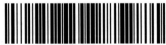

Made in the USA
San Bernardino, CA
18 June 2016